Functional Wellness: A Comprehensive Guide To Long-Term Fitness and Vitality

Terry M. Crafton

Table of Contents

Introduction

1.1 Definition and Significance of Functional Training

Functional training represents a dynamic and purposeful approach to fitness, centering its focus on movements that mirror real-life activities. In contrast to conventional workouts that isolate muscle groups, functional training emphasizes integrated exercises to enhance an individual's overall physical capabilities. It encompasses a spectrum of movements that emphasize coordination, balance, strength, and flexibility.

Key Elements of Functional Training:

1. Multi-Planar Movements: Functional training incorporates exercises that span various planes of motion—sagittal, frontal, and transverse. By engaging the body in diverse movement patterns, individuals develop a comprehensive fitness foundation, preparing them for the multidimensional challenges of daily life.

2. Integration of Core Muscles: Core strength is pivotal in functional training. Beyond targeting abdominal muscles, exercises engage the muscles of the lower back, hips, and pelvis. This holistic approach contributes to improved stability and balance.

3. Real-Life Application: The essence of functional training lies in its practicality. Exercises simulate activities encountered in daily life, such as bending, lifting, twisting, and reaching. Practicing these movements in a controlled environment translates to improved functional capacity and reduces the risk of injuries during routine tasks.

Significance of Functional Training:

1. **Improved Functional Capacity**:The core objective of functional training is to enhance an individual's ability to execute everyday activities more efficiently. From mundane tasks like carrying groceries to navigating complex movements, functional training contributes to a heightened functional capacity.

2. **Injury Prevention**: By targeting multiple muscle groups and promoting overall body strength, functional training serves as a preventive measure against injuries. Enhanced balance and coordination play a crucial role in reducing the risk of falls, especially among seniors.

3. **Enhanced** **Sports** **Performance**:
Athletes integrate functional training into
their routines to improve specific
movements pertinent to their sports. This
holistic approach fosters increased agility,
power, and overall athletic prowess.

4. Adaptability to Varied Fitness Levels:
Functional training is adaptable, catering
to individuals across different fitness
levels. Whether you're a beginner or a
seasoned fitness enthusiast, the versatility
of functional training makes it inclusive
and accessible to a diverse audience.

In essence, functional training transcends
the conventional fitness paradigm by
prioritizing movements that directly
impact daily life. Its holistic philosophy,
addressing strength, flexibility, and
coordination, positions it as an
indispensable component of a
comprehensive exercise regimen.

1.2 Understanding the Basics of Functional Exercises

Functional exercises serve as the cornerstone of a comprehensive fitness routine, distinguished by their focus on movements that directly translate to real-world activities. As we delve into the fundamentals of functional exercises, we uncover key principles that seamlessly align with the broader concepts discussed in the previous chapters.

Key Principles of Functional Exercises:

1. Natural Movement Patterns: Functional exercises embrace the innate movement patterns of the human body. These include fundamental actions like pushing, pulling, squatting, bending, and rotating—essentials in our daily lives. By adhering to these natural biomechanics, functional exercises contribute not only to improved mobility but also to the preservation of joint health.

2. Integration of Multiple Muscle Groups: Unlike traditional workouts, functional exercises are designed to engage various muscle groups simultaneously. This holistic approach not only fosters balanced muscle development but also fortifies overall functional strength, aligning seamlessly with the overarching goal of holistic wellness.

3. Focus on Stability and Balance: The incorporation of stability and balance into functional exercises becomes evident, mirroring the principles discussed in the earlier chapters. By emphasizing core stability and engaging stabilizer muscles, these exercises play a pivotal role in injury prevention and lay the groundwork for a resilient musculoskeletal system.

4. Versatility in Equipment and Settings: Functional exercises offer a level of adaptability that aligns harmoniously with the preceding discussions on progression and modifications. Whether using body weight, resistance bands, free weights, or specialized functional fitness equipment, individuals can tailor their workouts to their preferences, equipment availability, and fitness levels.

5. Progression through Movement Patterns: The progressive nature of functional training echoes the sentiments shared in the previous chapters about setting personalized fitness goals and gradually increasing intensity. Progressing through different movement patterns becomes a natural evolution, providing individuals with a structured path to advance their fitness journey.

Benefits of Incorporating Functional Exercises:

1. Enhanced Everyday Performance: The emphasis on natural movement patterns directly resonates with the objective of improving an individual's ability to perform daily tasks efficiently, a theme that aligns seamlessly with the goal of functional longevity.

2. Injury Prevention: The focus on stability, balance, and engagement of multiple muscle groups directly contributes to the prevention of injuries, reinforcing the importance of safeguarding one's well-being throughout the fitness journey.

3. Efficient Use of Time: The efficiency of functional exercises, engaging multiple muscle groups in each movement, dovetails with the tips for consistency provided in earlier chapters, making workouts not only effective but also time-efficient.

4. Adaptability to Varied Fitness Levels: Just as discussed in the progression and modification chapter, the adaptability of functional exercises allows individuals at different fitness levels to engage in workouts that suit their capabilities, fostering inclusivity and accessibility.

Chapter 1: The Foundation of Functional Longevity

In the pursuit of enduring well-being and a life filled with vitality, this chapter unfurls the profound interconnection between functional training and longevity. Positioned as a foundational cornerstone, it lays the groundwork for subsequent discussions, emphasizing the integral role that functional training plays in preserving physical independence, promoting holistic wellness, and fostering mental acuity across the spectrum of life.

1.1 Exploring the Interplay Between Functional Training and Longevity:

Beyond the mere extension of chronological existence, functional longevity emerges as a qualitative endeavor that seeks to optimize every facet of our existence. This section delves into the symbiosis between functional training and longevity, casting light on its transformative potential for individuals of all ages.

1. Holistic Wellness: Beyond the confines of traditional health metrics, functional longevity embraces a holistic ethos. It aspires not merely to prolong life but to enrich it, safeguarding essential elements such as mobility, flexibility, and mental well-being. The narrative unfolds a vision where well-being is not compartmentalized but rather, an interconnected tapestry of physical and mental vitality.

2. Adaptable Fitness Across Age Groups: The adaptability of functional training emerges as a unifying theme, making it an inclusive platform resonating with individuals across diverse age groups. From seniors seeking to fortify balance and mobility to younger enthusiasts laying the foundation for future well-being, functional training becomes a versatile and accessible fitness philosophy.

1.2 Benefits of Prioritizing Functional Movements for Long-Term Health:

Within this subsection, we embark on a nuanced exploration of the specific benefits that prioritizing functional movements bestows upon long-term health and vitality.

1. Joint Health: The intricate relationship between functional movements and joint health is unveiled. By aligning with natural movement patterns, functional exercises become an instrumental tool in promoting joint flexibility, mitigating the impact of aging, and fostering overall musculoskeletal resilience.

2. Cognitive Well-Being: The chapter delves deep into the cognitive benefits inherent in functional training. Beyond physical prowess, functional movements engage the mind, providing a holistic approach to preserving mental sharpness and agility. The interconnectedness of physical and cognitive well-being emerges as a cornerstone for a fulfilling and enduring life.

3. Independence in Daily Living: As life progresses through its various stages, the significance of maintaining independence in daily activities becomes paramount.

This section underscores how functional training cultivates the essential skills required for navigating daily tasks with autonomy and self-reliance.

4. Long-Term Sustainability: The narrative on the enduring nature of functional training is expanded further, positioning it not merely as a transient trend but as a lifelong companion in the pursuit of functional longevity. The sustainability of functional exercises over the long term becomes a defining factor in their effectiveness, underscoring the importance of a fitness philosophy that withstands the test of time.

As we draw the curtain on this foundational chapter, the intricate dance between functional training and longevity comes into sharper focus. The principles laid out here transcend conventional fitness paradigms, championing a holistic approach that resonates with individuals at every stage of life. This chapter sets the stage for a comprehensive exploration of how functional training intertwines with the fundamental aspects of longevity. By delving into the holistic benefits, adaptability, and enduring nature of functional movements, it propels us into a multifaceted journey towards sustained well-being across the entire spectrum of life.

Chapter 2: Functional Training

Ever wondered about those fitness courses you've come across? Let's break down functional training. Imagine it as the secret sauce for your everyday moves, like sitting, standing, reaching for stuff, or even pulling a car – all inspired by exercises like squats, presses, and pulls.

The cool thing? Functional fitness is like a chameleon, fitting into your day anytime, anywhere, and in any outfit. Whether you're into simple bodyweight exercises or spicing things up with cool adjustable dumbbells and stretchy bands, getting ready for functional strength training is your ticket to building muscles and boosting your heart health.

"Functional training isn't just about the gym," says the expert. "Nowadays, it's all about using bands, balls, ropes, kettlebells, sandbags, and even tires to get your body moving in different ways."

Picture functional training as a teamwork of muscles and joints – like a squat, where your hips, knees, and ankles gracefully bend and straighten. Your main muscle players, the glutes and quads, lead the show, with supporting roles from the hamstrings, calves, and erector spinae (they've got your back – literally). And we haven't even talked about your core muscles stepping up to the plate!

Functional training is like an art form outside the gym, inviting you to create a balanced dance of strength and flexibility in your body.

2.1. Core Principles of Functional Training

Functional training, often misconstrued, extends far beyond using gym equipment in unconventional ways. It is about replicating movements inherent in your sport or daily life. This chapter delves into the core principles that underpin functional training, providing a foundation for a holistic approach to fitness.

Defining Functional Training:

At its essence, functional training is not just about physical movements; it is a method that strengthens and conditions specific mechanical and energetic characteristics of the human body, aligning them with a targeted outcome. These principles are channeled through four pillars: locomotion, level changes, push and pull, and rotation.

Exploring Locomotion:

Irrespective of your activity, movement from point A to B is fundamental. Whether it involves skipping, jumping, sidestepping, or sprinting, single-leg movements take precedence. This section challenges the conventional use of squats and introduces the single-leg anterior reach as a more functional alternative.

Navigating Level Changes:

From low to high, the dynamics of movement change significantly. Staggered deadlifts, differing from the parallel stance of traditional deadlifts, become a functional choice when getting up from a fall or lifting an object. Using dumbbells or cables to vary the lift angle enhances the functionality of these exercises.

Engaging in Push and Pull Movements:

In daily life, pushing and pulling movements predominantly occur while standing, necessitating engagement of the core and specific muscle groups. The chapter advises on functional alternatives, suggesting standing cable presses over the traditional bench press for pushing strength and highlighting the effectiveness of bent-over rows as a superior functional pulling move compared to pull-ups.

Mastering Rotation:

Rotation demands a dual approach—acceleration and deceleration during sports activities like running or twisting. Developing rotational strength requires not only movement but also core stiffness. Traditional core exercises may fall short, and the chapter recommends twisting exercises using resistance bands or cables. A favorite, the band or cable rotation, is detailed as an ideal method for creating core strength with a dual-purpose focus.

2.2: Types of Functional Exercises for Comprehensive Fitness

Building upon the core principles discussed in the previous section, Chapter 2.2 explores various types of functional exercises tailored for comprehensive fitness. These exercises are designed to enhance not only specific muscle groups but also overall functionality, promoting a well-rounded approach to physical well-being.

Dynamic Movement Patterns:

Functional exercises are distinguished by their ability to replicate real-world movements. This section delves into dynamic movement patterns that engage multiple muscle groups simultaneously.

Exercises like medicine ball slams, woodchoppers, and kettlebell swings are explored for their efficacy in fostering coordination, strength, and flexibility.

Bodyweight Functional Training:

Functional fitness isn't always reliant on external weights. This part highlights the significance of bodyweight exercises, emphasizing movements that leverage your own body for resistance. Squats, lunges, push-ups, and planks are examined as fundamental bodyweight exercises that contribute to overall strength, stability, and endurance.

Balance and Stability Exercises:

Balance is a critical aspect of functional fitness, especially for seniors or those aiming to enhance stability. This section introduces exercises such as single-leg stands, stability ball exercises, and balance board activities. These exercises not only improve balance but also engage core muscles, contributing to overall stability.

Functional Training with Resistance Bands:

Resistance bands offer a versatile approach to functional training. They provide adjustable resistance levels and can be easily incorporated into various exercises. This part explores exercises like band pull-aparts, lateral walks, and resisted rotations, showcasing how resistance bands enhance muscle engagement and joint stability.

Agility and Speed Drills:

Functional fitness goes beyond strength; it encompasses agility and speed. Agility ladder drills, cone drills, and sprint variations are discussed to illustrate how incorporating these exercises can improve not only cardiovascular health but also enhance agility and quickness in daily activities.

Integrated Functional Workouts:

The chapter concludes by illustrating how to integrate different types of functional exercises into comprehensive workouts. Sample workout routines are provided, showcasing the combination of dynamic movements, bodyweight exercises, balance drills, resistance band training, and agility drills to create a well-rounded and effective functional fitness routine.

This section aims to equip readers with a diverse repertoire of functional exercises, offering a holistic approach to fitness that targets various aspects of physical well-being.

Chapter 3: Strength Training Recommendations

In Chapter 3, we delve into the crucial realm of strength training within the context of functional fitness. Understanding the importance of strength is paramount for overall functionality, and this chapter provides recommendations to tailor strength training to individual needs and abilities.

Importance of Strength Training:

Strength is the foundation of functional fitness. This section emphasizes the significance of strength training in enhancing muscle mass, bone density, and overall physical resilience. From improving daily activities to preventing injuries, the benefits of incorporating strength training into your routine are explored.

Functional Strength vs. Traditional Approaches:

Differentiating functional strength from traditional approaches is essential. The chapter compares functional strength, emphasizing real-world applications, with traditional strength training methods. It highlights the importance of engaging multiple muscle groups simultaneously to mimic the demands of daily life.

Tailoring Strength Training:

One size does not fit all in strength training. This part provides guidance on tailoring strength training routines to individual needs and abilities. Whether you're a beginner or an experienced fitness enthusiast, understanding your body and gradually increasing intensity is key to a sustainable and effective strength training program.

Functional Core Strength:

A strong core is central to functional fitness. This section explores exercises specifically designed to strengthen the core in ways that support overall functionality. Planks, anti-rotation exercises, and dynamic core movements are discussed to provide a well-rounded approach to building functional core strength.

Functional Movements for Everyday Activities:

The chapter showcases strength training exercises that directly translate into improved performance in daily activities. From lifting groceries to moving furniture, functional movements such as squats, deadlifts, and farmer's carries are dissected to highlight their relevance in enhancing daily functionality.

Adapting for Different Fitness Levels:

Fitness is a journey, and it's essential to adapt strength training to different fitness levels. This part offers modifications and progressions for various exercises, ensuring that individuals at different stages of their fitness journey can engage in effective and safe strength training tailored to their capabilities.

Progressive Overload for Functional Strength:

Progressive overload is a fundamental principle in strength training. This section explores how gradually increasing resistance, volume, or intensity is essential for continual improvement. By progressively challenging your muscles, you promote ongoing adaptations, leading to sustained gains in functional strength.

Balancing Muscular Imbalances:

Functional strength necessitates a balanced development of muscles to prevent imbalances that could lead to injuries. The chapter delves into strategies for addressing and correcting muscular imbalances, emphasizing the importance of targeting opposing muscle groups and addressing weaknesses to foster overall functional symmetry.

Functional Strength in Aging:

As we age, maintaining functional strength becomes increasingly crucial. This part discusses how strength training tailored to the needs of older adults can enhance mobility, bone density, and overall vitality. Exercises focusing on functional movements and joint flexibility are highlighted to support healthy aging.

Incorporating Functional Strength into Workouts:

The effectiveness of strength training lies in its integration into comprehensive workout routines. This section provides practical insights into seamlessly incorporating functional strength exercises into diverse workout plans. Whether you prefer full-body workouts or specific muscle group targeting, the chapter offers guidance on creating a well-rounded strength training routine.

Recovery Strategies for Strength Training:

Recovery is a vital component of any strength training program. This part explores strategies to optimize recovery, including proper nutrition, adequate sleep, and targeted stretching. Understanding the importance of recovery not only enhances the effectiveness of strength training but also prevents burnout and reduces the risk of injuries.

Monitoring and Adjusting Strength Training Programs:

No strength training program is static. Regular assessment and adjustment are key to long-term success. This section outlines how to monitor progress, identify areas for improvement, and make necessary adjustments to ensure ongoing effectiveness and prevent plateaus in functional strength development.

3.1 Importance of Strength Training for Overall Functionality

In this section, we delve into the cornerstone of functional fitness—strength training. Understanding the paramount importance of strength in the realm of overall functionality is key to unlocking a resilient, agile, and robust body capable of meeting the demands of everyday life.

Foundational Pillar of Functionality:

Strength is the bedrock upon which all functional movement patterns rest. Whether lifting, pushing, pulling, or simply navigating the challenges of daily activities, a robust foundation of strength underpins every motion. This part elucidates how strength serves as the fundamental building block for overall functionality.

Enhanced Muscle Mass and Metabolism:

Strength training goes beyond the immediate gains in muscle strength; it contributes significantly to increased muscle mass. More muscle mass not only elevates basal metabolic rate but also enhances the body's ability to burn calories at rest. This section explores how strength training, by fostering muscle growth, plays a pivotal role in maintaining a healthy body composition.

Bone Health and Density:

The importance of strength training extends to the skeletal system. Weight-bearing exercises stimulate bone formation and enhance bone density. This is particularly crucial in preventing osteoporosis and promoting overall bone health. The chapter details the role of strength training in fortifying the skeletal structure, ensuring longevity and resilience.

Joint Stability and Injury Prevention:

Functional movement relies on the stability of joints. Strength training targets the muscles surrounding joints, providing essential support and stability. By reinforcing these structures, individuals are better equipped to prevent injuries and navigate daily activities with reduced risk. This part emphasizes the symbiotic relationship between strength training, joint stability, and injury prevention.

Improving Functional Capacity:

Strength is the linchpin for expanding functional capacity. From the ability to carry groceries to the capacity for independent living, strength training directly correlates with improved functionality. The chapter explores how targeted strength exercises translate into enhanced performance in daily activities, fostering independence and quality of life.

Mitigating the Impact of Aging:

Aging often accompanies a natural decline in muscle mass and strength. Strength training emerges as a potent countermeasure. This section highlights how incorporating strength exercises into one's routine can mitigate the impact of aging, preserving muscle mass, bone density, and overall functionality well into the later stages of life.

Holistic Impact on Mental Health:

Beyond the physical benefits, strength training exerts a positive influence on mental well-being. This part explores the psychological aspects, discussing how the sense of accomplishment, improved self-esteem, and the release of endorphins contribute to a holistic enhancement of mental health through strength training.

Functional Independence:

Strength training lays the groundwork for functional independence. This section explores how building strength in various muscle groups directly translates into the ability to perform daily tasks without reliance on external assistance. From climbing stairs to lifting objects, the strength gained through targeted exercises empowers individuals to maintain autonomy in their activities.

Preventing Chronic Conditions:

The benefits of strength training extend to preventing chronic conditions. Maintaining muscular strength is linked to a reduced risk of chronic diseases such as diabetes, cardiovascular issues, and obesity. By actively engaging in strength training, individuals contribute to their long-term health and well-being, preventing the onset of debilitating conditions.

Enhanced Posture and Body Mechanics:

A robust musculoskeletal system, fostered through strength training, positively influences posture and body mechanics. This part delves into the connection between muscular strength and proper alignment, elucidating how strength training aids in maintaining good posture and optimal body mechanics. Improved alignment, in turn, reduces the risk of musculoskeletal issues.

Empowering Functional Longevity:

The section concludes by emphasizing how strength training is a key player in empowering functional longevity. As individuals age, the maintenance of strength becomes a linchpin for sustaining an active and fulfilling life. Strength training emerges as a reliable companion on the journey towards not just longevity but a life characterized by vitality and the ability to embrace new challenges.

3.2: Tailoring Strength Training to Individual Needs and Abilities

In this section, we navigate the nuanced terrain of tailoring strength training to individual needs and abilities. Recognizing that a one-size-fits-all approach may not be optimal, this chapter explores how customization can enhance the effectiveness and sustainability of strength training for diverse individuals.

Understanding Individual Goals:

The cornerstone of tailoring strength training lies in understanding individual goals. This part delves into the importance of clarifying personal objectives, whether they revolve around muscle gain, weight loss, enhanced athletic performance, or overall well-being. Tailoring strength training begins with aligning exercises with specific aspirations.

Assessing Fitness Levels:

A critical step in customization is assessing current fitness levels. The chapter discusses various assessment methods, from simple exercises to more advanced metrics, helping individuals gauge their strength, flexibility, and endurance. Understanding baseline fitness informs the design of a personalized strength training program.

Adapting for Beginners:

For beginners, embarking on a strength training journey can be intimidating. This section provides insights into easing newcomers into strength training, emphasizing proper form, gradually increasing intensity, and incorporating foundational exercises. Tailoring for beginners fosters a positive and sustainable introduction to strength training.

Progressive Overload Principles:

Tailoring strength training involves applying progressive overload principles. Exploring the concept of gradually increasing resistance, volume, or intensity, the chapter elucidates how this fundamental principle stimulates continual adaptations, promoting sustained gains in strength tailored to individual capabilities.

Modifying for Advanced Fitness Levels:

Advanced fitness enthusiasts require tailored strategies to continually challenge their bodies. The section delves into advanced strength training techniques, including periodization, varied rep ranges, and incorporating advanced exercises. Customization for advanced levels ensures ongoing progress and prevents plateaus.

Addressing Health Considerations:

Individual health considerations play a pivotal role in customization. This part explores how factors such as pre-existing conditions, injuries, or mobility limitations impact strength training. Tailoring exercises to accommodate health considerations ensures a safe and effective strength training experience.

Incorporating Preferences and Enjoyment:

Sustainability in strength training is closely linked to enjoyment. The chapter discusses how incorporating preferences, whether through choice of exercises, workout environment, or training style, contributes to long-term adherence. Tailoring strength training to align with individual preferences fosters a positive and enjoyable fitness experience.

Balancing Frequency and Duration:

Tailoring strength training involves finding the right balance between workout frequency and duration. The section provides insights into crafting a schedule that aligns with individual time constraints, ensuring that strength training remains a feasible and integral part of one's routine.

Customization for Age-Related Factors:

As individuals age, strength training requirements evolve. This part addresses how to tailor strength training programs to accommodate age-related factors such as joint health, recovery time, and overall fitness goals. Customization for different age groups ensures that strength training remains beneficial and accessible throughout the lifespan.

Individualizing Recovery Strategies:

Recognizing the individualized nature of recovery is crucial. The chapter explores tailored recovery strategies, including nutrition, sleep, and active recovery methods. Customizing recovery ensures that individuals optimize the benefits of strength training while minimizing the risk of burnout or overtraining.

Personalized Recovery Protocols:

An integral aspect of customization lies in tailoring nutrition to complement strength training. This section explores personalized nutritional considerations, such as caloric intake, macronutrient ratios, and hydration. Recognizing that individual bodies respond differently to dietary approaches, this chapter guides readers in aligning nutrition with their unique needs and goals.

Integrating Functional Movements:

Tailoring strength training involves integrating functional movements that align with daily activities. This part highlights the importance of incorporating exercises that mimic real-life motions, enhancing not only strength but also the practical applicability of the training. Functional movements contribute to improved functionality in day-to-day tasks, a key consideration in customization.

Personalized Recovery Protocols:

Recovery is a highly individualized aspect of strength training. The chapter delves into personalized recovery protocols, including strategies for managing muscle soreness, optimizing sleep patterns, and incorporating active recovery techniques. Tailoring recovery acknowledges the unique requirements of each individual, promoting sustained well-being throughout the training journey.

Psychological Considerations in Customization:

Beyond the physical realm, psychological factors play a pivotal role in customization. This section explores how individual motivations, mindset, and preferences influence the effectiveness of strength training. Tailoring approaches to align with psychological factors ensures a positive and empowering experience, fostering long-term adherence to strength training goals.

Tracking Progress and Adjusting Plans:

A key component of tailoring strength training involves continuous assessment and adjustment. The chapter provides insights into effective ways of tracking progress, whether through performance metrics, strength gains, or subjective feedback. Understanding how to adapt plans based on progress ensures that individuals stay engaged and motivated in their customized strength training journey.

Empowering Self-Efficacy:

Customization is a powerful tool in enhancing self-efficacy—the belief in one's ability to achieve desired outcomes.

This part explores how tailoring strength training empowers individuals by aligning exercises with personal preferences, abilities, and aspirations. Strengthening self-efficacy contributes to sustained commitment and enthusiasm for the strength training journey.

Building a Supportive Environment:

Creating a supportive environment is crucial for customization success. The section discusses the importance of social support, whether from friends, family, or a fitness community. Tailoring strength training to align with an individual's social context fosters a sense of belonging and encouragement, reinforcing the commitment to fitness goals.

Case Studies in Customization:

To provide practical insights, this chapter includes case studies illustrating successful customization strategies. These real-world examples demonstrate how individuals with varying needs and abilities tailored their strength training routines, showcasing the versatility and effectiveness of customization in achieving diverse fitness goals.

Chapter 4: Functional Movement Strategies for Daily Activities

In this chapter, we delve into practical and functional movement strategies tailored to enhance your daily activities. The goal is to integrate exercises seamlessly into your routine, promoting not only physical well-being but also improved efficiency and ease in performing everyday tasks.

Understanding Functional Movements:

Functional movements are those that mimic real-life activities and engage multiple muscle groups, promoting coordination and strength. This section introduces the concept of functional movements and their relevance to daily activities, laying the foundation for the strategies that follow.

Morning Mobility Routine:

Start your day with a set of mobility exercises designed to wake up your body and prepare it for the day ahead. This routine includes gentle stretches, joint movements, and balance exercises to promote flexibility and mobility, setting a positive tone for the day.

Incorporating Functional Exercises into Household Chores:

Discover how everyday chores can double as opportunities for functional exercises. From squats while loading the dishwasher to lunges while vacuuming, this section provides practical tips on infusing your household tasks with purposeful movements.

Desk-bound Mobility Breaks:

For those with sedentary jobs, this part offers a series of quick mobility breaks to combat the effects of prolonged sitting. Simple stretches, seated leg lifts, and shoulder rolls can be seamlessly incorporated into your work routine to enhance circulation and reduce stiffness.

Walking Techniques for Improved Functionality:

Walking is a fundamental daily activity, and optimizing your walking technique can have wide-ranging benefits. Explore tips on posture, stride length, and arm movement to make your walks not only enjoyable but also conducive to overall functional fitness.

Staircase Workouts for Strength and Endurance:

If you have access to stairs, they become a valuable resource for functional workouts. Learn how to leverage staircases for exercises that target leg strength, cardiovascular fitness, and balance, transforming a common feature into a fitness tool.

Functional Movements for Joint Health:

Maintaining joint health is crucial for daily mobility. This section introduces functional movements specifically designed to promote joint flexibility and strength. Exercises targeting the hips, knees, and shoulders contribute to overall joint well-being.

Dynamic Stretching Before Daily Activities:

Incorporating dynamic stretching into your pre-activity routine can enhance flexibility and reduce the risk of injuries. This part provides a set of dynamic stretches suitable for various daily activities, ensuring your body is primed for movement.

Evening Relaxation Routine:

Wrap up your day with a calming routine designed to promote relaxation and flexibility. Gentle stretches, deep breathing exercises, and mindfulness techniques contribute to winding down both physically and mentally.

Expanding on Daily Activity Integration:

Building upon the concept of incorporating functional movements into daily activities, this section provides additional examples and creative ideas. Whether it's turning household chores into full-body workouts or finding opportunities for functional movements during leisure activities, the goal is to make exercise seamlessly woven into the fabric of your daily life.

Seated Functional Exercises for Office Settings:

For those spending extended hours in an office setting, this part introduces a series of seated functional exercises. These exercises target core strength, posture, and flexibility, addressing the challenges of desk-bound routines and promoting an active approach to office-based fitness.

Functional Movement Breaks:

Recognizing the importance of taking breaks throughout the day, this section introduces the concept of functional movement breaks. Short, focused bursts of movement can reenergize both body and mind. From quick stretches to mini-workouts, these breaks aim to enhance productivity and well-being.

Adapting Functional Movements for Varied Fitness Levels:

Understanding that individuals have different fitness levels, this part explores how to adapt functional movements to suit varying capabilities. Whether you're a beginner or have advanced fitness, the exercises provided can be tailored to meet your current fitness level, ensuring inclusivity and accessibility.

Functional Movements for Enhanced Posture:

Good posture is integral to daily activities and overall well-being. This section focuses on functional movements that target core strength and postural muscles. By incorporating these exercises into your routine, you can work towards improving posture, reducing discomfort, and enhancing body awareness.

Integrating Functional Movements into Recreation:

Leisure activities present opportunities for functional movements. Whether you enjoy gardening, playing sports, or engaging in recreational hobbies, this part explores how to infuse these activities with purposeful exercises. This holistic approach ensures that your leisure time contributes to both enjoyment and physical fitness.

Addressing Common Daily Movement Challenges:

This section addresses common challenges individuals face in their daily movements. From addressing stiffness in the morning to combating fatigue in the afternoon, practical solutions and exercises are provided to overcome these challenges and maintain a consistent level of energy and vitality throughout the day.

Functional Movement Apps and Resources:

Explore the world of functional movement apps and resources designed to guide and motivate your daily exercise routine. From guided workout apps to movement tracking tools, this part introduces technological aids that can enhance your engagement with functional exercises.

Measuring Progress in Daily Functional Fitness:

Understanding the impact of functional movement strategies requires tracking progress. This section provides insights into how to measure improvements in strength, flexibility, and overall functional fitness. Establishing benchmarks and celebrating small victories contribute to the ongoing success of your daily functional fitness journey.

Encouraging Consistency through Habit Formation:

Consistency is key in reaping the benefits of functional movement strategies. This part explores the science of habit formation and provides practical tips for incorporating these exercises into your routine consistently. By establishing habits, you ensure that functional movements become an integral part of your daily life.

4.1: Integrating Functional Movements into Everyday Life

In this section, we delve into the practical aspects of seamlessly integrating functional movements into your everyday life. By making exercises an inherent part of your routine, you not only enhance physical fitness but also cultivate a mindful approach to movement in the context of your daily activities.

Functional Movements in Daily Chores:

Explore how routine household chores can be transformed into purposeful exercises. From squatting while picking up groceries to incorporating lunges while making the bed, this part provides insights into infusing functional movements into your daily chores, turning mundane tasks into opportunities for physical engagement.

Walking with Purpose:

Walking is a fundamental daily activity, and this section emphasizes walking with purpose. Whether it's focusing on maintaining proper posture, incorporating brisk intervals, or engaging your arms for a full-body workout, discover how to turn your daily stroll into a functional exercise that contributes to your overall well-being.

Active Commuting Strategies:

For those who commute regularly, this part explores ways to make your journey more active. From incorporating standing stretches on public transport to choosing stairs over escalators, these strategies ensure that your commute becomes an opportunity for light exercise, promoting circulation and energy.

Desk-bound Functional Movements:

Address the challenges of sedentary office work by introducing functional movements that can be seamlessly integrated into your workday. Simple exercises like seated leg lifts, desk push-ups, and shoulder rolls are presented to combat the negative effects of prolonged sitting and promote a more active work environment.

Functional Breaks During Screen Time:

Screen time often dominates our daily routines, and this section suggests incorporating functional breaks into prolonged periods of sitting. Quick stretches, eye exercises, and seated twists are introduced to counteract the sedentary nature of screen-related activities, fostering movement and reducing stiffness.

Functional Movements in Social Settings:

Discover how social gatherings and outings can become opportunities for functional movements. Whether it's incorporating standing stretches during a conversation or choosing activities that involve physical engagement, this part encourages a social environment that supports both connection and fitness.

Family Fitness Routines:

For families, creating fitness routines together enhances both physical health and bonding. This section provides ideas for family-friendly functional exercises that cater to different age groups. From backyard games to group activities, fostering a culture of family fitness becomes an enjoyable and shared experience.

Shopping as a Functional Exercise:

Turn your shopping trips into purposeful exercises by incorporating functional movements. This part suggests ways to engage your muscles while navigating the aisles, carrying bags, and loading your groceries. By making shopping an active experience, you contribute to your overall fitness without dedicating specific workout time.

Mindful Movement Practices:

Integrate mindfulness into your daily movements by adopting mindful movement practices. This section explores the benefits of being present in each motion, emphasizing the mind-body connection. By incorporating mindfulness, you not only enhance the effectiveness of your functional exercises but also cultivate a sense of tranquility.

Functional Movements in Outdoor Activities:

Explore how outdoor activities can be enriched with purposeful movements. Whether it's hiking, gardening, or playing recreational sports, this section suggests incorporating functional exercises that align with the natural flow of these activities. By making the most of the outdoor environment, you enhance both your fitness and connection with nature.

Functional Movements in Cooking and Meal Prep:

The kitchen becomes a dynamic space for functional movements as this part introduces exercises that can be seamlessly integrated into cooking and meal preparation. From standing balance exercises while stirring to incorporating squats while waiting, these movements contribute to your daily activity levels.

Stairs as a Functional Exercise Tool:

If you have stairs in your daily environment, this section explores leveraging them as a valuable tool for functional exercise. Stair climbing engages multiple muscle groups and enhances cardiovascular fitness. Learn different stair exercises and strategies for making stair use a purposeful part of your daily routine.

Functional Movements for Enhanced Posture at Work:

For those spending extended hours at a desk, maintaining good posture is crucial. This part introduces functional movements specifically aimed at improving posture during work hours. From seated stretches to midday posture resets, these exercises counteract the effects of prolonged sitting on posture and musculoskeletal health.

Functional Movements During Leisure Screen Time:

Even during leisure screen time, functional movements can be integrated to offset sedentary habits. This section suggests exercises such as seated leg extensions or neck stretches while watching TV or using digital devices. By incorporating movement into relaxation time, you promote a balance between screen-based entertainment and physical activity.

Functional Movements for Improved Sleep:

Explore how incorporating specific functional movements into your pre-sleep routine can contribute to better sleep quality. Gentle stretches, relaxation exercises, and mindful breathing techniques are introduced to create a bedtime ritual that not only relaxes the body but also enhances overall sleep hygiene.

Multi-tasking with Functional Movements:

Discover the art of multi-tasking by incorporating functional movements into activities that typically involve only one focus. Whether it's practicing balance exercises while brushing your teeth or doing calf raises while waiting for the kettle to boil, this section encourages efficiency in making the most of your time.

Functional Movements for Stress Reduction:

Recognizing the impact of stress on overall well-being, this part introduces functional movements that specifically target stress reduction. Exercises such as deep breathing, gentle stretches, and mindful movements contribute to creating moments of calm within your hectic schedule.

Daily Movement Journaling:

Consider keeping a daily movement journal to track your progress and reflect on the integration of functional movements into your everyday life. This section provides guidance on maintaining a simple journal that helps you stay accountable, set goals, and celebrate the successes in your journey towards a more active lifestyle.

Creating a Personalized Daily Movement Plan:

Tailor functional movements to your unique daily schedule by creating a personalized movement plan. This part offers practical tips on assessing your daily routine, identifying opportunities for movement, and developing a plan that aligns with your goals and preferences.

4.2: Enhancing Daily Activities through Purposeful Exercises

This section focuses on the intentional enhancement of daily activities through purposeful exercises. By infusing your routine with targeted movements, you not only amplify the efficiency of everyday tasks but also contribute to your overall physical well-being.

Functional Movements in Household Chores:

Explore how purposeful exercises can elevate the impact of household chores. From incorporating squats while loading the dishwasher to performing lunges while vacuuming, this part provides practical examples of how daily activities can become opportunities for muscle engagement and conditioning.

Efficient Movement Patterns:

Discover the concept of efficient movement patterns and how they can streamline daily tasks. This section emphasizes optimizing body mechanics during activities like lifting, reaching, and carrying to reduce the risk of strain or injury. Learn how simple adjustments in movement can significantly enhance the effectiveness of daily actions.

Balance and Stability Exercises:

Integrate balance and stability exercises into daily activities to enhance overall coordination. From standing on one leg while brushing your teeth to incorporating stability challenges while reaching for items, this part offers exercises that improve proprioception and support better control of movement.

Postural Awareness in Daily Tasks:

Develop postural awareness during routine activities to promote spinal health and muscle engagement. This section explores maintaining a neutral spine while sitting, standing, and bending to prevent undue stress on the back. By incorporating postural principles, you contribute to long-term musculoskeletal well-being.

Functional Movements in Work Tasks:

Apply purposeful exercises to enhance work-related tasks. Whether it's incorporating seated leg lifts during desk work or integrating standing stretches into short breaks, this part provides strategies for infusing movement into the workday. By optimizing movement at work, you support physical health and productivity.

Efficient Movement During Commuting:

Explore ways to make commuting more than just a means of transportation. This section suggests purposeful exercises like isometric contractions during transit or engaging your core while driving. By making your commute an active part of your day, you contribute to overall daily movement goals.

Purposeful Movements While Waiting:

Transform moments of waiting into opportunities for purposeful exercises. Whether it's calf raises while standing in line or seated stretches during a wait, this part encourages turning idle time into active moments. Learn how to make the most of these intervals to accumulate beneficial movement throughout the day.

Joint Mobility Exercises for Daily Flexibility:

Incorporate joint mobility exercises into daily routines to enhance flexibility. From gentle neck rotations to ankle circles, this section provides exercises that lubricate joints and promote overall mobility. By prioritizing joint health, you ensure a greater range of motion in daily activities.

Functional Movements in Leisure Activities:

Enhance leisure time with purposeful exercises that complement recreational activities. Whether it's integrating stretches into reading time or performing gentle exercises during screen-based entertainment, this part suggests ways to infuse movement into moments of relaxation.

Mindful Eating Practices:

Explore the concept of mindful eating as a purposeful exercise. This section encourages paying attention to body cues, taking breaks between bites, and incorporating subtle movements like seated twists. By fostering awareness during meals, you not only support digestion but also introduce purposeful movements.

Functional Movements in Social Gatherings:

Turn social gatherings into opportunities for purposeful exercises. This part suggests incorporating standing stretches, gentle movements, or even group activities during social events. By creating an environment that encourages both connection and movement, you contribute to a holistic approach to health.

Functional Movements for Improved Sleep:

Discover how incorporating specific functional movements into your pre-sleep routine can contribute to better sleep quality. Gentle stretches, relaxation exercises, and mindful breathing techniques are introduced to create a bedtime ritual that not only relaxes the body but also enhances overall sleep hygiene.

Multi-tasking with Functional Movements:

Explore the art of multi-tasking by incorporating functional movements into activities that typically involve only one focus. Whether it's practicing balance exercises while brushing your teeth or doing calf raises while waiting for the kettle to boil, this section encourages efficiency in making the most of your time.

Functional Movements for Stress Reduction:

Recognizing the impact of stress on overall well-being, this part introduces functional movements that specifically target stress reduction. Exercises such as deep breathing, gentle stretches, and mindful movements contribute to creating moments of calm within your hectic schedule.

Daily Movement Journaling:

Consider keeping a daily movement journal to track your progress and reflect on the integration of functional movements into your everyday life. This section provides guidance on maintaining a simple journal that helps you stay accountable, set goals, and celebrate the successes in your journey towards a more active lifestyle.

Creating a Personalized Daily Movement Plan:

Tailor functional movements to your unique daily schedule by creating a personalized movement plan. This part offers practical tips on assessing your daily routine, identifying opportunities for movement, and developing a plan that aligns with your goals and preferences.

Chapter 5: The Scale is Not a Useful Tool for Measuring Results

Challenge the conventional approach to measuring fitness progress by questioning the effectiveness of the scale. This chapter delves into the limitations of using weight as the primary metric for success and advocates for a more holistic and functional perspective on health and fitness.

Understanding the Scale's Limitations:

Explore the pitfalls of relying solely on weight as a measure of fitness. This section discusses how factors like water retention, muscle gain, and body composition can influence the numbers on the scale, often providing an incomplete and misleading picture of one's overall health and well-being.

Rethinking Traditional Measurement Metrics:

Encourage readers to shift their focus from weight-centric metrics to more meaningful indicators of progress. This part introduces alternative measurements such as body composition analysis, energy levels, and functional improvements as more accurate reflections of a person's fitness journey.

Emphasizing Functional Progress Over Scale Numbers:

Highlight the importance of functional progress as a true measure of fitness success. This section emphasizes how improvements in strength, flexibility, endurance, and overall functionality provide a more comprehensive and reliable gauge of one's well-being compared to arbitrary numbers on a scale.

Functional Fitness Assessments:

Introduce functional fitness assessments as valuable tools for tracking progress. This part discusses assessments that measure mobility, balance, and agility, providing a more insightful overview of an individual's fitness journey beyond what traditional scales can offer.

Case Studies:

Illustrate the shortcomings of relying solely on weight through real-life case studies. Share stories of individuals who experienced significant functional improvements without significant weight loss, demonstrating the importance of looking beyond the scale for a more accurate assessment.

Importance of Non-Scale Victories:

Celebrate non-scale victories as essential milestones in the fitness journey. This section explores achievements such as improved sleep, increased energy levels, enhanced mood, and a positive mindset as valuable markers of success that go beyond the numeric focus of traditional weight measurements.

Embracing a Mindful Approach:

Advocate for a mindful approach to health and fitness. This part encourages readers to tune into their bodies, listen to how they feel, and appreciate the positive changes happening internally, fostering a more sustainable and holistic mindset toward well-being.

Setting Meaningful Goals:

Guide readers in setting goals that extend beyond the scale. This section helps individuals identify personal, functional, and performance-based objectives, providing a roadmap for a fulfilling and purpose-driven fitness journey.

Tracking Functional Progress:

Offer practical advice on how to track functional progress effectively. Whether through journaling, incorporating fitness apps, or utilizing fitness assessments, this part equips readers with tools to monitor improvements that align with their unique fitness goals.

Understanding Body Composition:

Dive deeper into the concept of body composition and its significance in assessing fitness. This section explains how understanding the distribution of muscle, fat, and other tissues provides a more nuanced perspective on physical health compared to relying solely on total body weight.

Impact of Muscle Gain:

Explore the positive impact of muscle gain on overall health. This part breaks down the misconception that weight gain always equals fat gain, highlighting how building muscle can contribute to a leaner and healthier physique. Encourage readers to appreciate the role of muscle in functional fitness.

Debunking Weight Loss Myths:

Address common weight loss myths that perpetuate misconceptions about health and fitness. This section aims to debunk notions such as rapid weight loss equating to improved health, emphasizing the importance of sustainable and functional progress over quick fixes.

Functional Fitness Success Stories:

Share inspiring success stories of individuals who achieved remarkable functional fitness improvements without significant weight loss. These narratives serve as powerful examples of how focusing on functional goals can lead to transformative changes in overall well-being.

Educating on Metabolic Health:

Educate readers on the relationship between weight, metabolism, and overall health. Discuss how metabolic health, influenced by factors beyond weight, plays a crucial role in determining one's well-being. This section empowers individuals to prioritize metabolic health over arbitrary weight goals.

Mind-Body Connection:

Explore the mind-body connection and its impact on overall health. This part delves into how stress, mental well-being, and emotional health can influence physical health and, consequently, the effectiveness of fitness journeys. Encourage a holistic approach to well-being.

Functional Fitness Challenges:

Present challenges that focus on functional fitness rather than weight loss. This section introduces readers to practical challenges that emphasize improvements in strength, flexibility, and endurance. These challenges serve as motivational tools for those seeking a more functional and fulfilling fitness journey.

Integrating Functional Metrics:

Guide readers on integrating functional metrics into their fitness assessments. Whether it's tracking the ability to perform daily activities with greater ease or measuring improvements in specific exercises, this part provides tangible ways to shift the focus from the scale to meaningful functional indicators.

Community Support and Accountability:

Highlight the importance of community support in fostering a mindset shift away from the scale. Discuss how accountability partners, fitness communities, or support networks can contribute to a positive environment that encourages functional progress and celebrates diverse definitions of success.

Building a Resilient Mindset:

Empower readers with strategies to build a resilient mindset in their fitness journeys. This section offers tools for overcoming setbacks, embracing failures as learning opportunities, and cultivating a positive outlook that goes beyond the numbers on a scale

5.1: Rethinking Traditional Measurement Metrics

Challenge the established norms in fitness assessment by questioning the effectiveness of traditional measurement metrics. This chapter delves into the limitations of using weight as the primary metric for success and advocates for a more holistic and functional perspective on health and fitness progress.

Shortcomings of Traditional Metrics:

Discuss the limitations of traditional metrics such as body weight, BMI, and calorie counting. Explore how these metrics often fail to provide a comprehensive understanding of an individual's overall health and fitness level, neglecting crucial factors like body composition, muscle mass, and functional capabilities.

Body Composition as a Key Indicator:

Highlight the significance of body composition as a more accurate indicator of fitness. Explain how understanding the ratio of muscle to fat provides valuable insights into metabolic health, physical performance, and overall well-being. Encourage readers to prioritize body composition assessments over simplistic weight-focused metrics.

Functional Fitness Metrics:

Introduce the concept of functional fitness metrics that go beyond the conventional measurements. Discuss the importance of assessing strength, flexibility, agility, and endurance as integral components of a holistic fitness evaluation. Emphasize how these metrics align more closely with the goals of functional training.

Tailoring Metrics to Individual Goals:

Advocate for a personalized approach to fitness metrics based on individual goals. This section guides readers in selecting metrics that align with their unique aspirations, whether it's improving athletic performance, enhancing daily activities, or achieving specific functional milestones.

Mindful Eating and Intuitive Metrics:

Explore the role of mindful eating and intuitive metrics in fostering a healthier relationship with food. Discuss how paying attention to hunger cues, nourishing the body with nutrient-dense foods, and cultivating mindful eating habits can contribute to overall well-being, going beyond calorie-centric measurements.

Emotional and Mental Health Metrics:

Acknowledge the impact of emotional and mental health on overall well-being. Introduce the idea of incorporating emotional intelligence, stress management, and mental health assessments as essential metrics in the fitness journey. Highlight the interconnectedness of mental and physical health.

Holistic Wellness Metrics:

Promote a holistic approach to wellness by considering a broader spectrum of metrics. Discuss the inclusion of sleep quality, energy levels, mood, and overall life satisfaction as valuable indicators of a well-rounded and thriving lifestyle.

Encourage readers to view wellness as a multidimensional concept.

Progress Journals and Tracking:

Encourage the use of progress journals for tracking a diverse set of metrics. Provide guidance on creating personalized journals that encompass physical, emotional, and lifestyle metrics. Emphasize the value of reflection and self-awareness in the journey toward optimal health.

Educational Resources for Metric Understanding:

Provide recommendations for educational resources that empower individuals to understand and interpret various fitness metrics. This part equips readers with the knowledge needed to make informed decisions about their health and fitness, fostering a sense of autonomy and self-empowerment.

Exploring Holistic Wellness Metrics:

Delve deeper into the concept of holistic wellness metrics, emphasizing the interconnectedness of various aspects of well-being. Discuss how metrics such as sleep quality, stress levels, emotional balance, and life satisfaction contribute to a more comprehensive understanding of an individual's overall health. Encourage readers to broaden their perspective beyond physical metrics alone.

Customizing Metrics for Personal Goals:

Guide readers in tailoring metrics to align with their specific health and fitness objectives. Whether aiming for weight loss, muscle gain, improved athletic performance, or enhanced daily functionality, this section offers practical advice on selecting metrics that directly correlate with individual goals.

Utilizing Technology for Metric Tracking:

Introduce the role of technology in modern metric tracking. Discuss the benefits of fitness apps, wearables, and smart devices that allow individuals to monitor various aspects of their health and fitness journey. Emphasize how these tools can enhance awareness, motivation, and adherence to personalized metrics.

The Role of Professional Guidance:

Highlight the importance of seeking professional guidance in understanding and interpreting fitness metrics. Encourage readers to consult with fitness professionals, nutritionists, and healthcare providers to receive personalized insights into their unique metrics and to ensure a safe and effective fitness journey.

Empowering Mindful Eating:

Expand on the concept of mindful eating as a metric for nutritional well-being. Provide practical tips on developing mindful eating habits, recognizing hunger and fullness cues, and fostering a positive relationship with food. Showcase how mindfulness in eating can contribute to improved nutritional choices and overall health.

Incorporating Lifestyle Metrics:

Explore the inclusion of lifestyle metrics that go beyond traditional fitness assessments. Discuss how factors like daily movement, sedentary behavior, and recreational activities contribute to overall health. Guide readers in recognizing and optimizing lifestyle metrics for a more holistic approach to well-being.

Measuring Emotional Resilience:

Discuss the role of emotional resilience as a metric for mental well-being. Explore how individuals can assess their ability to cope with stress, setbacks, and challenges. Provide practical strategies for enhancing emotional resilience, emphasizing its significance in maintaining overall health and fitness.

Creating a Personalized Metric Toolkit:

Empower readers to create their personalized metric toolkit.

Offer a comprehensive guide on selecting, tracking, and interpreting metrics that align with individual values and aspirations. Encourage the integration of diverse metrics to paint a more accurate and personalized picture of health and fitness.

Promoting a Growth Mindset:

Encourage the adoption of a growth mindset when approaching metrics. Emphasize that metrics are tools for learning and improvement rather than strict measures of success or failure. Foster a positive and adaptive mindset that allows individuals to embrace challenges, learn from experiences, and continuously evolve on their fitness journey.

5.2: Emphasizing Functional Progress Over Scale Numbers

Shift the focus from conventional scale numbers to the significance of functional progress in the fitness journey. This chapter advocates for a holistic approach that prioritizes improvements in functional capabilities over simplistic weight-oriented metrics.

Challenges with Scale Numbers:

Discuss the limitations of relying solely on scale numbers for gauging fitness success. Address the common pitfalls, such as overlooking muscle gain, neglecting body composition changes, and fostering an unhealthy fixation on weight reduction. Highlight how scale numbers often fail to capture the broader spectrum of improvements.

Defining Functional Progress:

Introduce the concept of functional progress, emphasizing advancements in strength, flexibility, mobility, and overall functionality. Illustrate how these aspects contribute to improved daily life, enhanced athletic performance, and a more resilient and capable body.

Encourage readers to redefine their definition of success in the fitness journey.

Functional Fitness Benchmarks:

Present a range of functional fitness benchmarks that extend beyond weight-related goals. Discuss how achieving milestones like mastering specific exercises, increasing stamina, or improving joint mobility can serve as powerful indicators of progress. Showcase the versatility of functional benchmarks in assessing overall fitness.

Measuring Strength and Endurance:

Explore the importance of measuring strength and endurance as key components of functional progress. Provide insights into how advancements in lifting heavier weights, performing more repetitions, or sustaining physical activities for longer durations reflect improvements in muscular and cardiovascular fitness.

Assessing Flexibility and Mobility:

Highlight the role of flexibility and mobility assessments in tracking functional progress. Discuss how increased range of motion, improved joint flexibility, and enhanced mobility contribute to better movement patterns, reduced injury risk, and overall functional well-being.

Functional Movement Patterns:

Discuss the significance of mastering functional movement patterns as a measure of progress. Explore how exercises that mimic real-life movements, such as squats, lunges, and twists, can translate into improved performance in daily activities. Emphasize the connection between functional movements and enhanced quality of life.

Adapting Workouts for Functional Gains:

Provide practical advice on adapting workout routines to focus on functional gains. Discuss the incorporation of compound exercises, full-body movements, and varied workout modalities that prioritize functional fitness. Guide readers in designing workouts that align with their individual functional goals.

The Role of Consistency:

Emphasize the role of consistency in achieving functional progress. Discuss how regular, sustainable efforts contribute to long-term improvements in functional capabilities. Encourage readers to embrace the journey and celebrate incremental functional gains as markers of success.

Celebrating Non-Scale Victories:

Encourage readers to celebrate non-scale victories as powerful motivators. Explore the emotional and psychological impact of acknowledging and appreciating improvements in functional abilities. Foster a positive mindset that recognizes the value of the entire fitness journey, beyond numerical measurements.

Progress Tracking Beyond Weight:

Encourage readers to diversify their approach to progress tracking beyond weight-related metrics. Discuss the relevance of body measurements, changes in clothing fit, and visual progress photos as alternative ways to measure the impact of fitness efforts. Highlight how these indicators provide a more comprehensive view of physical transformation.

Holistic Wellness Metrics:

Integrate the concept of holistic wellness metrics into the discussion, emphasizing how improvements in sleep quality, stress management, and overall well-being contribute to functional progress. Illustrate the interconnectedness of various lifestyle factors and their impact on both physical and mental fitness.

Functional Progress in Daily Activities:

Explore how functional progress directly translates into improved performance in daily activities. Discuss real-life examples of individuals who have experienced enhanced ease in tasks such as lifting groceries, climbing stairs, or playing with children due to their functional fitness improvements. Reinforce the idea that true success extends beyond the gym.

Adaptive Exercise Modifications:

Provide guidance on adaptive exercise modifications that accommodate individual needs and challenges. Discuss how individuals with different fitness levels, body types, or health conditions can tailor their workouts to emphasize functional progress. Encourage inclusivity in fitness by showcasing diverse approaches to functional training.

Functional Progress Assessments:

Introduce various assessments for tracking functional progress. Discuss the use of fitness tests, movement screenings, and functional evaluations to quantify improvements in specific areas. Illustrate how these assessments can serve as benchmarks for setting and achieving functional fitness goals.

The Mind-Body Connection:

Explore the mind-body connection in the context of functional progress. Discuss how a positive mindset, mental resilience, and emotional well-being contribute to overall functional fitness. Emphasize that a holistic approach to health includes nurturing both physical and mental aspects.

Educational Resources for Functional Fitness:

Provide recommendations for educational resources that empower individuals to understand the principles of functional fitness. Suggest books, articles, and online platforms that offer insights into the science and application of functional training. Equip readers with the knowledge needed to make informed decisions about their fitness journey.

Community Support and Accountability:

Highlight the role of community support and accountability in fostering functional progress. Discuss the benefits of joining fitness communities, participating in group workouts, or seeking guidance from fitness professionals. Illustrate how a supportive environment can enhance motivation and adherence to functional fitness goals.

Overcoming Setbacks and Challenges:

Acknowledge that setbacks and challenges are inherent in any fitness journey. Provide strategies for overcoming obstacles and staying resilient in the pursuit of functional progress. Share stories of individuals who have navigated setbacks and emerged stronger, reinforcing the idea that resilience is a crucial aspect of the journey

Chapter 6: Create Your Personal Fitness Journey

Embarking on a personal fitness journey is a transformative and empowering decision. This chapter is your guide to crafting a fitness plan that resonates with your goals, preferences, and lifestyle. It's not just about exercise; it's a holistic approach to enhancing your overall well-being. Let's delve deeper into the key elements that will shape your unique fitness journey.

•Setting Personalized Fitness Goals:

1. Define Your Objectives:
   - Begin by clearly defining your fitness objectives. Whether it's weight loss, muscle gain, improved endurance, or overall well-being, understanding your specific goals forms the foundation of your personalized fitness journey.

2. SMART Goals:
   - Dive into the concept of SMART goals—Specific, Measurable, Achievable, Relevant, and Time-bound. Learn how to formulate goals that are realistic, trackable, and tailored to your unique aspirations.

•Designing a Sustainable Fitness Plan:

1. Fitness Preferences:

- Explore various types of exercises and activities to identify what resonates with your preferences. Whether it's strength training, cardio, yoga, or a combination, a sustainable plan aligns with personal enjoyment.

2. Balancing Workouts:

- Emphasize the importance of a balanced workout routine. Include components for cardiovascular health, strength building, flexibility, and relaxation. A well-rounded approach addresses different aspects of fitness and reduces monotony.

3. Progressive Overload:

- Understand the principle of progressive overload—gradually increasing intensity to stimulate continual adaptation. Design workout plans that challenge you without risking injury.

4. Consistency and Variety:

   - Stress the value of consistency while incorporating variety. Maintain regular workout schedules while exploring diverse activities to prevent boredom and keep motivation high.

5. Adaptability:

   - Acknowledge that life is dynamic, and fitness plans should be adaptable. Adjust your routines based on changing circumstances, ensuring long-term sustainability.

•Balancing Nutrition and Exercise:

1. Nutritional Goals:

   - Discuss the synergy between nutrition and exercise. Guide you in setting nutritional goals that complement your fitness objectives, whether it's weight management, muscle building, or overall health.

2. Hydration:
   - Highlight the importance of hydration in supporting physical activity. Provide practical tips for maintaining adequate water intake throughout the day and during workouts.

3. Nutrient-Rich Choices:
   - Encourage a focus on nutrient-dense foods that fuel your body for optimal performance. Discuss the significance of a well-balanced diet rich in proteins, carbohydrates, fats, vitamins, and minerals.

•Prioritizing Recovery:

1. Sleep and Rest:
   - Highlight the role of sleep and rest in the recovery process. Discuss the impact of quality sleep on overall well-being and

muscle recovery. Provide strategies for improving sleep hygiene.

2. Active Recovery:

- Introduce the concept of active recovery, incorporating light exercises, stretching, or activities like yoga on rest days. Emphasize that recovery is an integral part of fitness progress.

•Building a Support System:

1. Accountability Partners:

- Encourage you to enlist support from friends, family, or workout buddies. Discuss the benefits of accountability partners in staying motivated and committed to fitness goals.

2. Online Communities:

- Explore the role of online fitness communities and social media groups. Discuss how sharing experiences, seeking advice, and celebrating achievements with like-minded individuals can enhance motivation.

•Reflection and Adaptation:

1. Regular Reflection:
   - Stress the importance of regular self-reflection on the fitness journey. Assess your progress, celebrate achievements, and identify areas for improvement.

2. Adapting Goals:
   - Discuss the possibility of adapting fitness goals based on changing circumstances, achievements, or evolving aspirations. Flexibility in goal-setting contributes to sustained motivation.

As you navigate your personal fitness journey, remember that it's a dynamic and ongoing process. Embrace the uniqueness of your path, stay adaptable, and celebrate the positive changes happening in your life. Your commitment to health and well-being is a lifelong investment, and every step forward is a victory. Best of luck on your journey!

6.1: Setting Personalized Fitness Goals

Setting personalized fitness goals is the cornerstone of a successful and fulfilling fitness journey. In this section, we'll delve into the process of defining objectives that are specific to you, providing direction and purpose to your endeavors. Let's embark on the first step towards a healthier and happier you.

1. Define Your Objectives:
- The journey begins with a clear understanding of what you want to achieve. Whether it's weight loss, muscle gain, enhanced endurance, or overall

well-being, define your objectives with clarity. Take the time to reflect on what truly matters to you.

2. SMART Goals:

- Introduce the SMART criteria—Specific, Measurable, Achievable, Relevant, and Time-bound. Apply these principles to your fitness goals. For instance, instead of a vague goal like "lose weight," make it specific, measurable, achievable within a set timeframe, and relevant to your overall well-being.

3. Long-Term and Short-Term Goals:

- Distinguish between long-term and short-term goals. Long-term goals provide a broader perspective, while short-term goals break down the journey into manageable steps. This approach allows you to celebrate achievements along the way and stay motivated.

4. Consider Your Lifestyle:

- Tailor your fitness goals to your lifestyle. Recognize the demands of your daily life, work, and personal commitments. Setting realistic goals that align with your schedule increases the likelihood of adherence.

5. Personal Values and Motivation:

- Align your fitness goals with your personal values and motivations. Understand why these goals are essential to you. Whether it's improved health for your family, increased energy for work, or a personal achievement, connecting your goals to your values enhances their significance.

6. Account for Variety:

- Embrace variety in your fitness goals. Include different dimensions such as cardiovascular health, strength training, flexibility, and mental well-being. A well-rounded approach ensures comprehensive fitness and prevents monotony.

7. Gradual Progression:

- Plan for gradual progression. Avoid setting overly ambitious goals that may lead to burnout or injury. Progress at a pace that challenges you without overwhelming your current fitness level.

8. Adaptability:

- Acknowledge that circumstances change. Your goals should be adaptable to life's fluctuations. Be prepared to modify your objectives based on evolving priorities, unforeseen challenges, or new opportunities.

Setting personalized fitness goals is a dynamic process that requires introspection, planning, and adaptability. As you define your objectives, remember that they are uniquely yours, designed to enhance your well-being and align with your aspirations. Embrace this step with enthusiasm, and let your goals be a source of inspiration on your journey to a healthier and happier lifestyle.

6.2: Designing a Sustainable Fitness Plan for Long-Term Success

Congratulations on defining your personalized fitness goals! Now, let's transition to the next crucial step—designing a sustainable fitness plan. This section will guide you in crafting a holistic approach that ensures long-term success, incorporating balance, adaptability, and enjoyment.

1. Fitness Preferences:
   - Explore various types of exercises to identify what resonates with you. Whether it's strength training, cardio, yoga, or a combination, a sustainable plan aligns with activities you genuinely enjoy. This

ensures consistency and increases the likelihood of adherence.

2. Balancing Workouts:
   - Emphasize the importance of a balanced workout routine. Incorporate components for cardiovascular health, strength building, flexibility, and relaxation. A well-rounded approach addresses different aspects of fitness, reducing the risk of overtraining and monotony.

3. Progressive Overload:
   - Introduce the principle of progressive overload. Gradually increase the intensity of your workouts to stimulate continual adaptation. This not only enhances physical performance but also prevents plateaus and keeps your fitness journey dynamic.

4. Consistency and Variety:

- Stress the value of consistency while incorporating variety. Maintain regular workout schedules while exploring diverse activities to prevent boredom and keep motivation high. Consistency builds habits, and variety keeps your fitness routine exciting.

5. Adaptability:
   - Acknowledge that life is dynamic, and fitness plans should be adaptable. Encourage the ability to adjust your routines based on changing circumstances, ensuring long-term sustainability. Adaptability is key to overcoming challenges and staying committed.

•Balancing Nutrition and Exercise:

6. Nutritional Goals:
   - Discuss the synergy between nutrition and exercise. Guide readers in setting nutritional goals that complement their fitness objectives, whether it's weight

management, muscle building, or overall health. A well-fueled body supports optimal performance.

7. Hydration:
   - Emphasize the importance of hydration in supporting physical activity. Provide practical tips for maintaining adequate water intake throughout the day and during workouts. Hydration is essential for overall health and exercise performance.

8. Nutrient-Rich Choices:
   - Encourage a focus on nutrient-dense foods that fuel the body for optimal performance. Discuss the significance of a well-balanced diet rich in proteins, carbohydrates, fats, vitamins, and minerals. Nutrition plays a vital role in achieving fitness goals.

•Prioritizing Recovery:

9. Sleep and Rest:

- Highlight the role of sleep and rest in the recovery process. Discuss the impact of quality sleep on overall well-being and muscle recovery. Provide strategies for improving sleep hygiene to support your fitness journey.

10. Active Recovery:

- Introduce the concept of active recovery. Incorporate light exercises, stretching, or activities like yoga on rest days. Emphasize that recovery is an integral part of fitness progress and contributes to overall well-being.

•Building a Support System:

11. Community Engagement:

- Discuss the importance of community engagement, whether through local fitness classes, online forums, or social media groups. A supportive community can provide motivation, inspiration, and a sense of belonging.

12. Accountability Partnerships:

- Explore the benefits of accountability partnerships. Encourage readers to involve friends, family, or workout buddies to share the journey, celebrate successes, and overcome challenges together.

•Reflection and Adaptation:

13. Regular Self-Reflection:

- Stress the importance of regular self-reflection on the fitness journey. Encourage readers to assess progress, celebrate achievements, and identify areas for improvement. Reflection enhances mindfulness and awareness.

14. Adapting Goals:

- Discuss the possibility of adapting fitness goals based on changing circumstances, achievements, or evolving aspirations. Flexibility in goal-setting contributes to sustained motivation and a positive mindset.

Designing a sustainable fitness plan is a pivotal step toward long-term success. By balancing workouts, prioritizing nutrition, emphasizing recovery, building a support system, and embracing adaptability, you're creating a framework that goes beyond exercise—it's a lifestyle. As you embark on this journey, remember that each decision contributes to your overall well-being. Here's to your sustained success and a healthier, happier you!

Conclusion: Navigating Your Holistic Fitness Journey

As we conclude this exploration into the realm of holistic fitness, it's time to reflect on the insightful journey we've embarked upon together. From understanding the fundamental principles of functional training to delving into personalized fitness goals and sustainable plans, our endeavor has been a comprehensive guide to cultivating a healthier, fitter, and more fulfilling life.

In Chapter 1, we unraveled the profound connection between functional training and longevity. We witnessed the transformative benefits of prioritizing movements that echo the rhythms of everyday life, paving the way for sustained health over the long term.

Chapter 2 immersed us in the core principles of functional training, elucidating how these principles are the bedrock for comprehensive fitness. From locomotion to push and pull, the understanding of functional exercises has expanded, providing a diverse toolkit for optimizing the body's mechanical and energetic characteristics.

The significance of strength training took center stage in Chapter 3. We recognized its pivotal role in enhancing overall functionality and explored the art of tailoring strength training to individual needs and abilities. A personalized approach emerged as the key to unlocking one's full physical potential.

Chapter 4 transported us into the fabric of daily life, unveiling strategies to seamlessly integrate functional movements into our routines. From purposeful exercises to enhancing daily activities, we discovered that fitness is not confined to the gym but is a dynamic part of our every waking moment.

In Chapter 5, we challenged the conventional metric of the scale, urging a shift towards rethinking traditional measurement metrics. Emphasis was placed on the journey's progress, celebrating the functional advancements rather than being confined to numerical benchmarks.

Our journey culminated in Chapter 6, where the spotlight was on creating a personal fitness odyssey. From setting personalized goals to designing sustainable plans for long-term success, we navigated the intricacies of crafting a fitness journey that aligns with individual aspirations and preferences.

As you stand at the intersection of knowledge and action, armed with the insights gathered in these chapters, the path forward is yours to forge. Embrace the ongoing nature of your fitness expedition, adapting goals as needed and relishing in the continuous journey towards health and well-being.

In closing, remember that your pursuit of holistic fitness is not just a physical endeavor; it's a holistic transformation. Every stride you take, every goal you achieve, and every obstacle you overcome contributes to the narrative of your well-being. As you navigate the dynamic landscape of health, may your steps be purposeful, your goals inspiring, and your commitment unwavering.

Congratulations on reaching this juncture of your fitness odyssey. The road ahead is filled with opportunities for growth, and the pages of your health and well-being story are waiting to be written. Here's to your continued success, vitality, and the flourishing chapters that lie ahead.

Wishing you a future filled with health, happiness, and a lifelong commitment to your holistic fitness journey.

Cheers to a Vibrant and Fulfilling Life!

www.ingramcontent.com/pod-product-compliance
Lightning Source LLC
Chambersburg PA
CBHW070847260726
48661CB00004B/1280